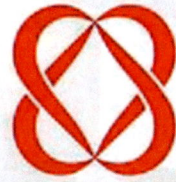

LEGACY
HEART CARE

Health & Wellness
Program Essentials

*Name:*_____   *Start Date:*_____

My Notes

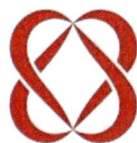

Welcome!

Welcome to Legacy Heart Care! During the next two months, our goal is to provide you not only the best EECP experience possible but also one that is tailored to your unique health needs. Here, we take a comprehensive and personalized approach to your health and wellness, where our mission is to *empower you to reach your optimal health by helping you take control of your health, while simultaneously providing a supportive environment for you to achieve your personal wellness goals.*

During your time here, you will be undergoing daily EECP treatments. At the same time, you will take part in Legacy's Health & Wellness program—a program designed to help you...

1. *Achieve* **your personal healthy living goals**
2. *Maximize* **the benefits of your EECP treatments**

Each week, you will meet with your clinical director, one-on-one, to address any health concerns and to discuss wellness topics that are important to you--these can range from nutrition to physical fitness, stress management to the management of your specific chronic conditions. Working together, you will focus on making personal, achievable goals that in turn lead to lifelong, healthy living habits that will improve your overall health and enrich your sense of well-being.

In this *Program Essentials* booklet, you will find valuable health tools that are designed to complement your book, *Being Empowered for a Healthy Heart.* Together, these program components will help you maximize the benefits of your EECP treatments as well as guide you toward your personal health and wellness goals. We encourage you to take advantage of these materials and to utilize the health management tools included within.

On behalf of all of us here, we are very excited to have you at Legacy Heart Care, and we look forward to joining you on this upcoming journey to greater health and wellness!

Sincerely,

The Legacy Heart Care team

My Notes

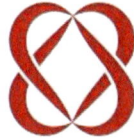

Table of Contents

Quick Symptom Checker

EVERY DAY

EVERY DAY

- Weigh yourself in the morning before breakfast. Write it down. Compare your weight today to your weight yesterday.

- Keep the total amount of fluids you drink to only 6 to 8 glasses each day. (6-8 glasses equals 1500-2000 mL or 48-64 oz)

- Take your medicine exactly how your doctor said.

- Check for swelling in your feet, ankles, legs, and stomach.

- Eat foods that are low in salt or salt-free.

- Balance activity and rest periods.

Where Are You Today?

GREEN SAFE ZONE

ALL CLEAR - This zone is your goal!

Your symptoms are under control. You have:

- No shortness of breath.
- No chest discomfort, pressure, or pain.
- No swelling or increase in swelling of your feet, ankles, legs, or stomach.
- No weight gain of more than 4 lbs (2 kg) over 2 days in a row or 5 lbs (2.5 kg) in 1 week.

YELLOW CAUTION ZONE

CAUTION - This zone is a warning

Call your Health Care provider (eg. Doctor, nurse) if you have any of the following:

- You gain more than 4 lbs (2 kg) over 2 days in a row or 5 lbs (2.5 kg) in 1 week.
- You have vomiting and/or diarrhea that lasts more than two days.
- You feel more short of breath than usual.
- You have increased swelling in your feet, ankles, legs, or stomach.

- You have a dry hacking cough.
- You feel more tired and don't have the energy to do daily activities.
- You feel lightheaded or dizzy, and this is new for you.
- You feel uneasy, like something does not feel right.
- You find it harder for you to breathe when you are lying down.
- You find it easier to sleep by adding pillows or sitting up in a chair.

Healthcare Provider: _____ **Phone Number:** _____

RED DANGER ZONE

EMERGENCY - This zone means act fast!

Go to emergency room or call 9-1-1 if you have any of the following:

- You are struggling to breathe.
- Your shortness of breath does not go away while sitting still.
- You have a fast heartbeat that does not slow down when you rest.
- You have chest pain that does not go away with rest or with medicine.
- You are having trouble thinking clearly or are feeling confused.
- You have fainted.

My Personal Health Plan

What I hope to achieve with my EECP treatments

❖

My top health concerns

1.
2.
3.
4.

My personal healthy living goals

1.
2.
3.
4.

My main barriers to achieving goals

1.
2.
3.
4.

Do you use smoke tobacco? ☐ Yes   ☐ No

It has been shown that people who quit smoking often experience even more benefits from EECP.

Would you like some useful information on how to cut down or quit smoking?   ☐ **Yes** ☐ **No**

Being Empowered for a Healthy Heart

Book Progress

Chapter	Topic	Date Completed	Notes
1	Being an Empowered Patient		
2	Action Planning		
3	Getting the Most Out of Medications		
4	The Heart Healthy Diet		
5	Exercising with Heart Conditions		
6	Taking Control of Angina		
7	Taking Control of High Blood Pressure		
8	Taking Control of Diabetes		
9	Taking Control of Heart Failure		
10	Taking Control of Chronic Lung Disease		
11	Taking Control of Chronic Pain		
12	Stress Management		
13	Relaxation Techniques		
14	Managing Depression		
15	Preventing Heartburn		
16	Fighting Fatigue		
17	Insomnia & Sleeping Problems		
18	Urinary Incontinence		
19	Maintaining Intimacy		
20	Preventing Holiday Illness		
21	Being Empowered to Quit Smoking		
22	Staying Motivated		

- Week 1 -

My Action Plan

This week, I will...

Confidence Level _____

☐ Check when completed!

Book Chapters	Discussion Topic
☐ Chapter 1: Being an Empowered Patient	
☐ Chapter 2: Action Planning for Success	
☐ Chapter 3: Getting the Most Out of Your Medications	

Step Count

M_____ T_____ W_____ TH_____ F_____ S_____ S_____

Personal Notes

- Week 2 -

My Action Plan

This week, I will...

Confidence Level _____

☐ Check when completed!

Book Chapters	Discussion Topic
☐ Chapter 4: Eating for Heart Health	
☐ Chapter 5: Physical Activity & Exercise	
☐ Chapter 6: Taking Control of Angina	

Step Count

M_____ T_____ W_____ TH_____ F_____ S_____ S_____

Personal Notes

- Week 3 -

My Action Plan

This week, I will...

Confidence Level _____   ☐ Check when completed!

Chapters for Next Week	Discussion Topic
☐ **Chapter 7: Taking Control of High Blood Pressure**	
☐ **Chapter 8: Taking Control of Diabetes** *(if applicable)*	
☐ **Chapter 9: Taking Control of Heart Failure** *(if applicable)*	

Step Count

M_____ T_____ W_____ TH_____ F_____ S_____ S_____

Personal Notes

- Week 4 -

My Action Plan

This week, I will...

Confidence Level _____   ☐ Check when completed!

Chapters for Next Week	Discussion Topic
☐ **Chapter 10: Taking Control of Lung Disease** *(if applicable)*	
☐ **Chapter 11: Taking Control of Chronic Pain** *(if applicable)*	
☐ **Chapter 12 & 13: Stress Management & Relaxation Techniques**	

Step Count

M_____ T_____ W_____ TH_____ F_____ S_____ S_____

Personal Notes

- Week 5 -

My Action Plan

This week, I will...

Confidence Level _____

☐ Check when completed!

Chapters for Next Week

☐ Chapter 14: Managing Depression *(optional)*

☐ Chapter 15: Preventing Heartburn

☐ Chapter 16: Fighting Fatigue

Discussion Topic

Step Count

M_____ T_____ W_____ TH_____ F_____ S_____ S_____

Personal Notes

- Week 6 -

My Action Plan

This week, I will...

Confidence Level _____

☐ Check when completed!

Chapters for Next Week

☐ Chapter 17: Insomnia & Sleeping Problems

☐ Chapter 18: Urinary Incontinence *(optional)*

☐ Chapter 19: Maintaining Intimacy *(optional)*

Discussion Topic

Step Count

M_____ T_____ W_____ TH_____ F_____ S_____ S_____

Personal Notes

- Week 7 -

My Action Plan

This week, I will...

Confidence Level _____   ☐ Check when completed!

Chapters for Next Week	Discussion Topic
☐ Chapter 20: Preventing Holiday Illness	
☐ Chapter 21: Being Empowered to Quit Tobacco *(optional)*	
☐ Chapter 22: Staying Motivated	

Step Count

M_____ T_____ W_____ TH_____ F_____ S_____ S_____

Personal Notes

- Week 8 -

My Action Plan

This week, I will...

Confidence Level _____   ☐ Check when completed!

Chapters for Next Week	Discussion Topic
☐	
☐	
☐	

Step Count

M_____ T_____ W_____ TH_____ F_____ S_____ S_____

Personal Notes

My Medication List

Name:
Birth Date:
Phone Number:
Emergency Contact:

Home Address

Date	Medication Name	Dose	Directions for Taking	Reason for Taking	Notes / Doctor's Name

Date	Medication Name	Dose	Directions for Taking	Reason for Taking	Notes / Doctor's Name

Salt Tracker

Daily Sodium Limit: _____   **Date:** _____

Meal	Food	Sodium (mg)	Notes
Breakfast			
Lunch			
Dinner			
Snacks			
Total Sodium			

Date: _____

Meal	Food	Sodium (mg)	Notes
Breakfast			
Lunch			
Dinner			
Snacks			
Total Sodium			

Date: _____

Meal	Food	Sodium (mg)	Notes
Breakfast			
Lunch			
Dinner			
Snacks			
Total Sodium			

Fitness Log

Date/Time	Activity	Duration or Amount of Activity	How I Felt Afterwards	Notes

Fitness Log

Date/Time	Activity	Duration or Amount of Activity	How I Felt Afterwards	Notes

Angina Log

Date/Time	Angina Rating (1-10)	Suspected Trigger	Duration	What I Did to Make It Go Away	Notes

Angina Log

Date/Time	Angina Rating (1-10)	Suspected Trigger	Duration	What I Did to Make It Go Away	Notes

Blood Pressure Log

Date/Time	Blood Pressure AM | PM		Heartrate	How I Was Feeling

Date/Time	Blood Pressure AM | PM		Heartrate	How I Was Feeling

Diabetes Meal Planner

Recommended Carbohydrate Servings Per Meal
Women: 3 - 4   Men: 4 - 5

Date:_____

Meal	Food	Carbohydrate Servings	Grams of Carbohydrate
	Example: 1 Cup oatmeal	*2*	*30 g*
Breakfast			
Lunch			
Dinner			
Snacks			
Daily Total			

Date_____

Meal	Food	Carbohydrate Servings	Grams of Carbohydrate
Breakfast			
Lunch			
Dinner			
Snacks			
Daily Total			

Date_____

Meal	Food	Carbohydrate Servings	Grams of Carbohydrate
Breakfast			
Lunch			
Dinner			
Snacks			
Daily Total			

Weight Tracker

Date/Time	Weight	Symptoms	Notes

Date/Time	Weight	Symptoms	Notes

Stress Journal

Date/Time	Cause of Stress	How It Made You Feel (Physically & Emotionally)	Coping Strategy

Date/Time	Cause of Stress	How It Made You Feel (Physically & Emotionally)	Coping Strategy

Monthly Stress Reduction Tracker

Month _____

	1	2	3	4	5	6	7	8	9	10	11	12	13	14	15	16	17	18	19	20	21	22	23	24	25	26	27	28	29	30	31
STRESS LEVEL																															
Very High																															
High																															
Medium																															
Low																															
RELAXATION TECHNIQUE USED																															
Breath deeply, slowly																															
Meditate or pray																															
Stay in the moment																															
Stay Positive																															
Reach out to others																															
Laugh out loud, use humor																															
Play soothing music																															
Move your body, walk, dance																															
Go outside																															
Make a gratitude list																															
STRESS LEVEL AFTER TECHNIQUE																															
Very High																															
High																															
Medium																															
Low																															

Monthly Stress Reduction Tracker

Month _____

	1	2	3	4	5	6	7	8	9	10	11	12	13	14	15	16	17	18	19	20	21	22	23	24	25	26	27	28	29	30	31
STRESS LEVEL																															
Very High																															
High																															
Medium																															
Low																															
RELAXATION TECHNIQUE USED																															
Breath deeply, slowly																															
Meditate or pray																															
Stay in the moment																															
Stay Positive																															
Reach out to others																															
Laugh out loud, use humor																															
Play soothing music																															
Move your body, walk, dance																															
Go outside																															
Make a gratitude list																															
STRESS LEVEL AFTER TECHNIQUE																															
Very High																															
High																															
Medium																															
Low																															

Quick Relaxation Techniques

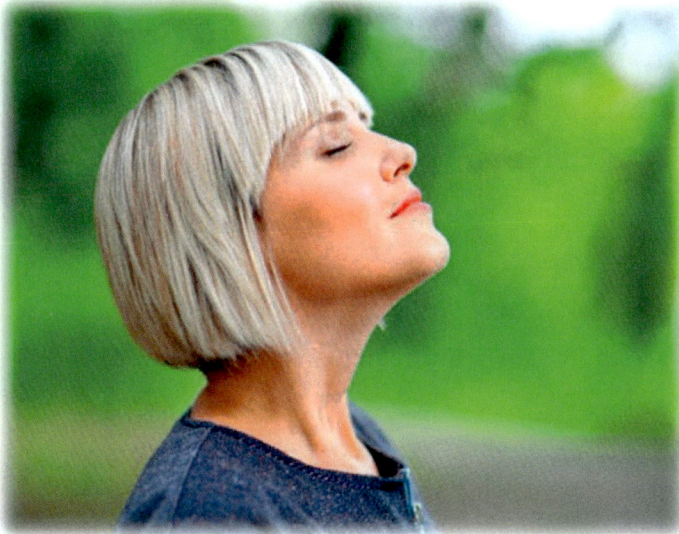

While it is ideal to have a regular time set aside for relaxation, sometimes one just needs a break from the stresses of a busy day—in the middle of the day.

These mini-relaxation techniques are powerful stress busters that you can reach for anytime. Whether you're preparing for an important meeting, stuck in traffic, or in the middle of an uncomfortable situation—these exercises can be a fast and effective tool to help you achieve a relaxed state so that you can confidently face the stresses of the day. So go ahead—take some time to try them all to see which ones work best for you.

Breathing Techniques

These techniques counteract the effects of stress by **slowing the heart rate** and **lowering blood pressure**.

Step 1	Step 2	Step 3	Step 4	Step 5	Step 6
Sit in a Comfortable Position	Close Your Eyes	Breathe In Slowly and Count to Five	Feel Your Belly Fill with Air	Breathe Out Slowly Through Your Mouth	Repeat This Cycle Five Times

Focused Breath (30 seconds)

1. **Sit back** in a comfortable position.
2. Begin breathing **slowly** and **naturally**.
3. Quietly whisper **"I am"** as you breathe in and **"at peace"** as you breathe out.
4. **Repeat** this several times.
5. **Feel** your entire body relax into the support of your chair.

Deep Breathing (30 seconds)

1. **Sit back** in a comfortable position.
2. **Place one hand on your belly,** so you can feel it rise and fall with each breath.
3. **Breathe in slowly** through your nose.
4. **Hold the air** within your lungs for 4 seconds.
5. Pucker your lips, and **slowly exhale** through your mouth for 6 seconds.
6. **Repeat** several times

Tense & Release (2 min)

When we hold onto worries and stress, our muscles unconsciously tighten. Most of the time we don't even notice how tense we are--until the tension leads to aches, pain, and exhaustion.

This technique is about **helping your body let go of all that tension**. By first tensing your muscles and then loosening them, you force your body to release the stresses of the day.

How to do it:

1. **Sit or lie** in a comfortable position.

2. While taking a deep breath in, **tense your entire body** by squeezing every muscle you can--from your face down to your toes.

3. **Hold this tension and your breath** for 5 seconds.

   ➤ Notice the heaviness and tightness

4. **While exhaling, relax all of your muscles**, imagining all the built-up tension and stress in your body melting away into the ground

   ➤ Notice the lightness of your body

5. As you take **slow, deep breaths**, **continue focusing** on how soft your muscles are and how relaxed you feel.

6. Continue this until you feel completely relaxed.

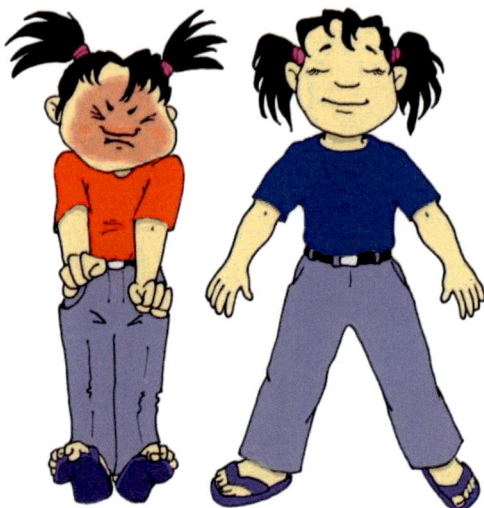

Mindfulness (1 min)

Rather than worrying about the future or dwelling on the past, the act of mindfulness switches the focus to what's happening **right now**, allowing you to be **fully engaged in the present moment**.

Use this technique when you are at work, home, or even when you are doing activities such as walking, exercising, or eating…whenever you need a dose of calmness.

How to do it:

1. The first time you try this, get in a **comfortable position**—sitting in a chair or cross-legged on the floor.

2. **Focus on an aspect of your breathing**:

   ➤ The sensation of air flowing into your nostrils and out of your mouth

   ➤ Your belly rising and falling

3. Now, begin to **widen your focus**:

   a. The sounds you **hear**

   b. The sensations you **feel**

   c. The objects you **see**

4. **Embrace** and **consider** each thought or sensation without judging it good or bad.

5. If your mind starts to race, **return your focus** to your breathing and repeat the exercise.

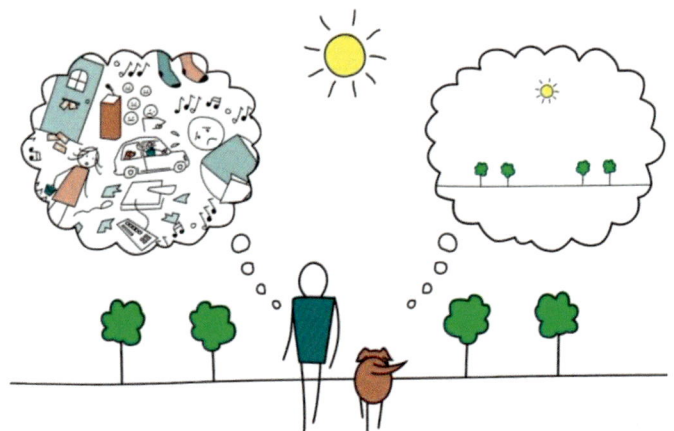

Mind Full, or Mindful?

Seated Stretches

SHOULDER CIRCLES

1. In a seated position, place your fingertips on your shoulders.

2. Circle your shoulders 15 times in a forward direction, then 15 times in the opposite direction.

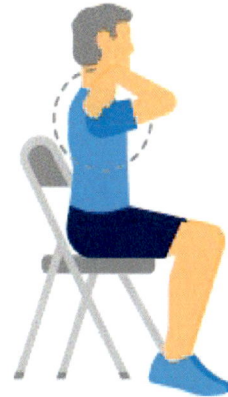

UPPER BACK STRETCH

1. Relax your shoulders with your arms resting by your side.

2. Extend your arms forward at shoulder height and grab one hand with the other and push outwards while pulling your back and shoulders forward.

3. Hold for 10 seconds and release. Repeat.

CHEST STRETCH

1. Relax your shoulders with your arms resting by your side.

2. Pull your arms back while grabbing one hand, keeping both hands down near your buttocks.

3. Pull your shoulders back and hold for 10 seconds and release. Repeat.

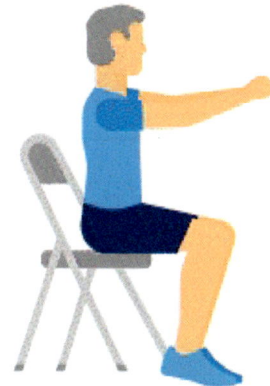

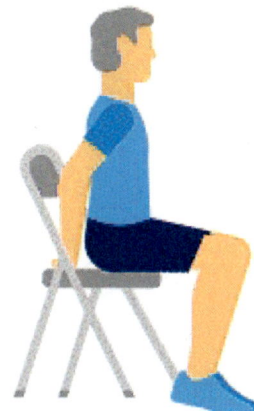

SIT AND REACH

1. Sit at the edge of a chair and extend your legs forward with your knees slightly bent.

2. Keep your heels on the floor and toes pointed toward the ceiling.

3. Extending both arms in front of you, reach down and touch your toes, slowly bending at the waist. (Stop when you feel resistance. Do not bounce up and down.)

4. Hold for 10 seconds before returning to your resting position. Repeat.

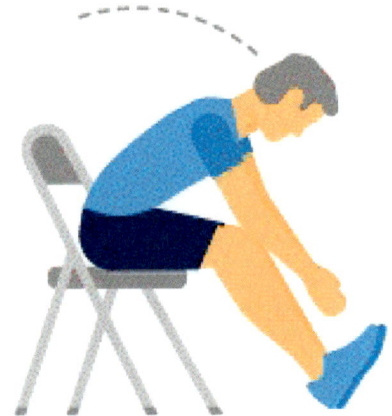

NECK STRETCH

1. In a seated position with your feet flat on the floor, slowly tilt your head to your right shoulder.

2. Hold this position and extend your left arm to the side and downward at waist level.

3. Release, then repeat on the left side.

4. Repeat twice on each side.

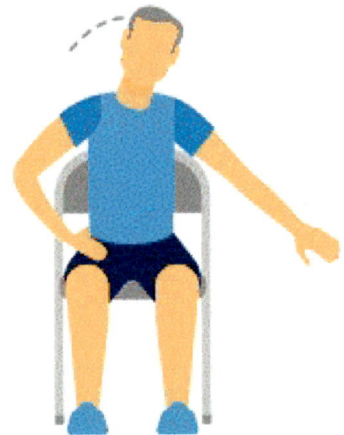

HAND STRETCH

1. Begin seated with your hands stretched out in front of you, palms facing each other.

2. Open both hands to spread your fingers apart, then close your hands.

3. Repeat 10 times.

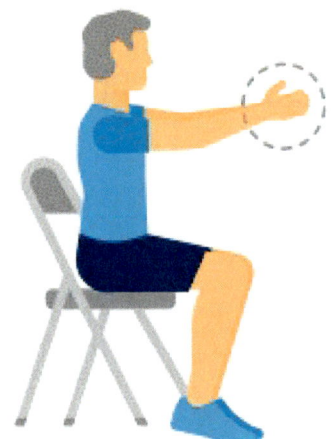

Seated Exercises for Strengthening

FRONT ARM RAISES

1. Begin seated, holding a ball in both hands with your palms facing each other.

2. Extend your arms forward so the ball rests on your legs, with your elbows slightly bent.

3. Slowly raise your arms to lift the ball to shoulder level, then lower back down, taking about 3 seconds to raise and lower.

4. Repeat 10-15 times.

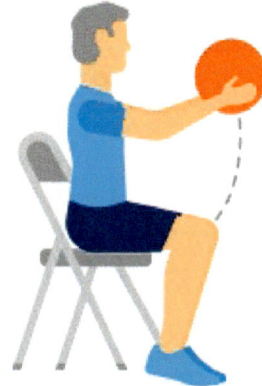

SHIN STRENGTHENER

1. Begin seated on the edge of a chair with legs extended, heels on the floor and knees slightly bent.

2. Point your toes downward, then flex upward.

3. Do 15 repetitions, then relax.

4. Repeat with 15 more repetitions.

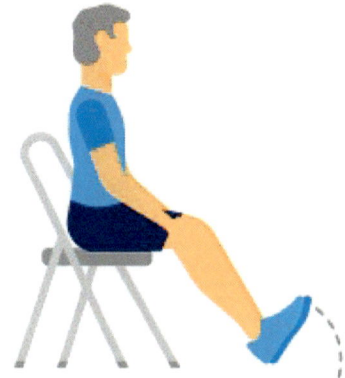

SIDE BENDS

1. Sit on a chair with your feet flat on the floor.

2. Place one hand behind your head and the other arm stretched out to one side.

3. Lean over to the side as if reaching toward the floor.

4. Return to the starting position, keeping your feet flat on the floor. Repeat 5 times on each side

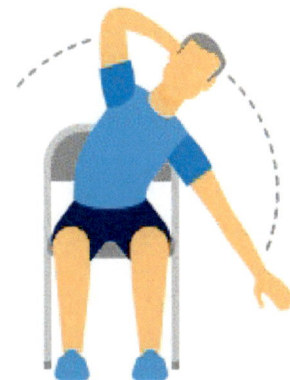

KNEE LIFTS

1. Begin seated on a chair.

2. Slowly draw one of your knees towards your body until it touches your chest.

3. Perform 15 to 20 repetitions for each leg.

4. Slowly work up to doing 3 sets at a time.

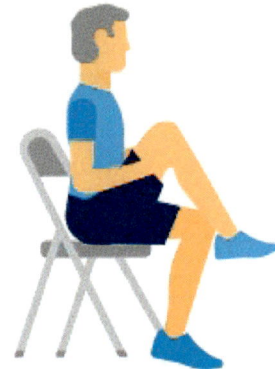

BICEP CURLS

1. Begin sitting in a chair with one dumbbell (or anything weighted—even a canned soup!) in each hand, with your palms facing up, keeping your elbows close to your sides.

2. Bend your arm at the elbow to lift one dumbbell almost to your shoulders, without moving your elbows away from your side.

3. Do 10 to 12 repetitions with each arm.

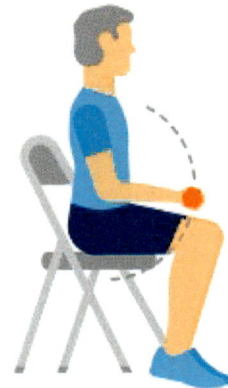

TUMMY TWISTS

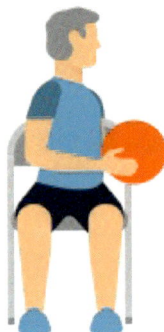 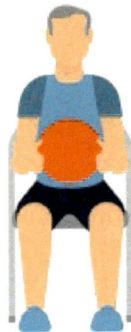 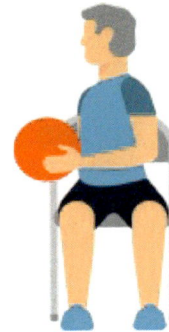

1. Facing forward in a seated position, hold a ball with both hands close to your stomach, your elbows slightly bent.

2. Slowly rotate your upper body to the right as much as you comfortably can while keeping the rest of your body stable.

3. Return to the center and repeat on the left. Complete 8 twists per side.

My Health Journal

Made in the USA
Lexington, KY
12 January 2019